HOW TO SUCCESSFULLY QUIT SMOKING
Proven steps to quit smoking without willpower

ALLEN COLLINS

COPYRIGHT

Copyright © 2021 by ALLEN COLLINS: All rights reserved. This book or any portion thereof may not be reproduced or used in any manner whatsoever without the express written permission of the author except for the use of brief quotations in a book review.

INTRODUCTION page 5

CHAPTER ONE page 9

Why is Quitting so Hard? 9

CHAPTER TWO page 13

How to Identify Your Smoking Triggers 13

CHAPTER THREE page 19

How to Manage Cigarette Cravings 19

CHAPTER FOUR page 25

Think Positive 25

CHAPTER FIVE page 29

Get Moving 29

CHAPTER SIX page 35

Your Personal Quit Smoking Plan 35

CHAPTER SEVEN page 41

Foods to Help Quit Smoking 41

CHAPTER EIGHT page 45

Preventing Weight Gain after You Stop Smoking 45

CHAPTER NINE page 51

What to Do if You Slip or Relapse 51

CHAPTER TEN page 57

Helping a Loved One to Stop Smoking 57

CONCLUSION page 63

INTRODUCTION

From habits we tend to create a consistent pattern of activities, sometimes we find ourselves entrapped into habits that we find really difficult to come out from, by this I mean addiction. Habits become an addiction when they become habitual in our daily routine. Some people are addicted to habits that do not affect their health but might affect their emotional wellbeing, while others have addictions that are bad for their health.

I once saw a man smoking and he was crying, I later found out that his smoking addiction had made him lose good relationships because his addiction endangered his loved ones. The goal of this book is to help people who have smoking addiction quit smoking and live a more green and serene life.

In 0.41 seconds, a search on 'how to quit smoking' on Google returns over 173 million responses. This represents the litany of information available on how-to when it comes to quitting smoking. With millions of answers, however, those in need of the information can only have it muddled and unseparated. Even if you continuously overdrink water, it has a side effect which is 'hyponatremia'; the same applies to smoking which is formed as a habit. When smoking is not stopped, it makes one prone to life-claiming diseases, complications, and dysfunctions. However, to break a smoking habit, capnophobia (fear of smoking) won't work; neither will fear-mongering of smoking effects work. Thus, a practicable habit-breaking strategy is needed to quit smoking. These strategies are what we'll go through together as we move into chapters of this book.

You may be wondering how it is possible to quit an addiction that has lingered for years, not to worry follow me through this journey as I help you find a sustainable solution to smoking addiction.

Something I always say is this, never give up on yourself there is still good to be done in 60 minutes, and luckily we have 24 hours every day to become a better version of ourselves.

Take back your life as we journey in this book on how to quit smoking addiction, it begins with the can-do mindset, let's dive in and become smoke-free.

CHAPTER ONE
Why is Quitting so Hard?

The human brain is wired to enjoy good moments, more reasons why we tend to create memorable moments because we love to enjoy the pleasures of life. At birth we have zero worries and no traits attached to us, everything we learnt or would learn in our lifetime could be linked to our associations and environment. In this chapter, we need to understand the origin of smoking, before a problem is solved the root cause has to be analysed.

Understanding the reason behind why quitting smoking is very difficult could serve as a pointer to the right direction. Listed below are a few reasons why our fear of addiction takes hold on us.

Addictive pleasure: The question that bothers your mind is, 'why is it hard to quit?' You certainly have one time or the other looked around for information on quitting smoking or might have even decided to quit only for you to pick up smoking days after that decision. The question that reverberates is, why so hard? Experts in nicotine research, have explained why it's difficult to quit smoking. They termed nicotine as being addictive, this means that there is a major link between pleasure and addiction. Nicotine is found in cigarettes and is more addictive than cocaine or heroin. Nicotine is just as hard as or harder to quit than heroin but people find it hard to believe it while others don't recognize it. Experts have carefully established the fact that nicotine stimulates pleasure through dopamine, this explains why you can find it tough to quit – everyone enjoys pleasurable feelings.

Habitual Repetition: Quitting smoking is hard because it's a habit. Just like Rome wasn't built in a day, breaking a habit doesn't happen overnight. Because breaking a habit demands intentional determination, readiness and efforts to drive the will, you can get scared of how long it can take to stop; won't I start gaining weight if I stop; won't I lose weight; do you really think I can do it? These reoccur when it's time to break that habit of smoking. You know how it feels when you're moved to smoke. Something triggers you to take a cigarette this could happen when you are lost in thought. The trigger is a stimulus, and because the brain receives the incoming sign as a rush of pleasure, you find yourself repeating the habit and longing to smoke every time if not daily. Neurologists from MIT have established the nexus between smoking and the smoking habit; when the brain receives a stimulus (a sign to light a cigarette), the smoking that follows becomes a habit. It is hard to quit because neurons located in the habit formation region fire at the beginning of a new behaviour occurs and then fire again once the behaviour is finished.

CHAPTER TWO
How to Identify Your Smoking Triggers

There is always something that brings back those flashback memories that ignites that addiction you are willing to quit, to find the solution the question is this, do you know that trigger that makes you want to smoke? If no please observe yourself and your environment and list out those triggers, If you must have figured out your smoking triggers stay tuned to the chapter where I would help you create a quit smoking plan.

In ensuring that the decision to quit works, you need to identify what triggers you to smoke. To some, it is the feelings that follow taking a caffeine contained drink, feeling of isolation, after completing a meal, finishing a coffee, in between tasks, a negative happening or a sight of a cigarette pack or an ashtray. Psychologists have confirmed that due to human differences, different things stimulate actions in people. This is why Mr A may be triggered by the sight of a cigarette while Mr B is triggered by tobacco smell or that of cigarette. A common trigger is the expectation of pleasure. The brain becomes conditioned in a way that not smoking feels like bondage and smoking is loosening from the contraption. It is essential to know what signals the brain to be in hasty demand for nicotine which many people may find difficult to control when stimulated. It's like taking fire out of a roof. Knowing your trigger makes you work to stamp it out gradually; like avoiding a gathering of other smokers if you're pushed by cigarette flavour, please keep all ashtrays and cigarettes' packs away from where they can be seen.

Smoking cravings would come now and then, which would make you want to have a taste, a smell, wanting to hold something or put something in your mouth. Sometimes you are just very restless that you find it hard to quit smoking, not to worry there are a few practical guides you can adopt to distract your brain from smoking addiction. Let us identify the smoking triggers and how to cope with them in this chapter.

Copying with emotional triggers: You have to understand your emotions, please take time to study yourself and know those things that could give you addictive pleasure as we talked about earlier in this book. Human emotions ranges from anxiety, happiness, loneliness, boredom, satisfaction, stress, and a whole lot of others. What you need to discover is how emotions affect your goal to quit smoking. For instance, what happens before you have the urge to smoke, you need to figure this out and prepare an escape route. The best way to overcome your trigger emotionally and physically is first becoming self-aware, this helps you think things through or talk to yourself. Know or discover what you need to do to bring calm to emotional triggers, a little recommendation here could be; exercising, taking pictures of nature, listening to a mind awareness podcast, enjoying a piece of calming music, learning a new dance routine or try some self-discovery exercise on some friends and family. Along these lines of doing some relaxing activities could help you cope with some emotional triggers.

Copying with social triggers: Sometimes we learn certain habits when we are socializing with other people, it is said by psychology experts that our brain tends to imitate the character traits of those we spend 60% - 80% of our time with. Socializing with people is good but if we further analyze what happens in social gatherings it could serve as a pointer to the way people act the way they do, it is just a way our brain imitates traits. Social triggers sometimes arises from association. For instance, going to a club or seeing someone else smoke could bring a flashback to your brain to create the urge to smoke despite your plans to completely quit the act of smoking. To deal with social triggers that could cause you to desire smoking you need to quit places where smoking takes place, also try to keep your distance from those who smoke this would help reduce every sort of things that could cause social triggers for you. Being social is cool but if it is the cause of your smoking triggers please keep a distance. Also tell your buddies that smoke that you are keeping a distance because you plan on completely quitting smoking, when this works for you, there is a possibility that your social buddies might also quit smoking.

Coping with pattern triggers: I was reading an article sometimes ago on how to rewire the brain to break out from habits that have created schedules or patterns in our everyday lives and I discovered that the factor of fear is the reason why we feel that it is difficult to achieve a certain milestone. There are a million ways to quit smoking but If you are in doubt or fearful, it becomes difficult to break out from the pattern of smoking. A quick exercise you can do to discover pattern triggers to smoking is to know: What you are always doing while smoking? Connect the dots and find a quick replacement. Let me give an example: Drinking alcohol and smoking. Find out what you do while smoking and find a quick fix. I would recommend busy hand therapy. Some busy hand exercise could be playing an instrument, riding a bike, writing a book, cleaning your home, crotchet knitting, create your juice recipe or play a ball sport.

CHAPTER THREE
How to Manage Cigarette Cravings

It's one thing to feel heavy about the dark side of smoking. Imagine what happens to your lungs, heart and other organs when you smoke non-stop. It's another thing to overcome the desire to smoke. When the feelings come, you're moved to light up. It takes efforts to repel the cravings. Or not repel but finding an alternative activity as a response to the stimulus (smoke signal).

It's important to know how to cope with nicotine. You have to always remember that the dopamine that comes from nicotine which equally gives you pleasure is attached to the possibilities of causing blood clots, plaque forms on the artery wall (atherosclerosis), dizziness, disturbed sleep, indigestion and heart-related diseases. To avoid these consequences you have to focus on quitting smoking. Things that can help is to remain committed to the plan to quit smoking. You can find alternative and healthy sources of pleasure or opt for alternative therapies. Although nicotine dependence stimulates pleasure, aids memory and concentration, you have to keep in mind the long term effects which include heart, hormonal and gastrointestinal problems.

The struggles on letting go of the cravings to smoke, even though you tried on countless times to quit, would always return some people to smoking when the urge to smoke comes. The smoking struggle is hard, tough as some people have these for years with back and forth thoughts on the decision to quit. Your brain could finally accept the fact that you are addicted to smoking but the body might have several constraints to totally eliminate smoking habits. It is all about nicotine, nothing more nothing less. Every craving and desire you have for the little devils is just a want for the nicotine. Therapy to quit smoking is not just about little pep talks, it should involve activities like cycling, photography, jogging and others when the craving kicks again. It is possible to finally get free from addictions when you know that you are in control of your life there should be no hidden or intentional desire to smoke. As long as blood runs through your veins, the craving for smoking will come but having in place the right tasks or strategies will keep away the urge and activate your decision to quit smoking. Manage your smoking habit with these few therapies listed below, please remember the goal of this book is to help you find the solution that works best for you. You have to make that effort to find out what's the best remedy for you and stick to a 30-day non-smoking plan.

Substitution therapy: Give your mouth something to do to bite on try: sugarless gum or hard sweets, carrots, celery, nuts or sunflower seeds — something crunchy and interesting. Try a nasal splash or inhaler, chew sugar-free gum as these substitution therapies could help reduce your smoking cravings. These short-acting treatments are by and large safe to use in blend with some meds recommended by your physician.

Trigger Avoidance: Whenever the desire comes, always remember this motto: Keep away from triggers. You may be enticed to have only one cigarette, don't trick yourself into accepting that you can stop there. Usually, having just one prompts another and this could ruin your plan to quit smoking. Try not to set yourself up for a smoking backslide. If you generally smoke while chatting on the phone, for example, keep a pen and paper close by to involve yourself with doodling instead of smoking. Desires to smoke could arise from any circumstances that brings a reminder to your brain, for example, at gatherings or bars, or while feeling focused or tasting coffee. Recognize your trigger circumstances and have an arrangement set up to maintain a strategic distance from them totally or overcome them without giving smoking a thought.

Postponement: If you have a feeling that you will yield to your cravings to smoke, try this quick fix; remind yourself to hold on for 10 minutes and afterwards plan something to really occupy yourself for that timeframe. Something interesting you need to try is to get a Zero smoke zone logo or visit a place that has that sign as this would trick your brain to comply with your decision of postponement.

Energy Burn: Get physical, a little work can help occupy you from the desire to smoke. Control is key you need to learn how to diminish and dominate the power smoking has over your life. A short eruption of actual work like running all over the steps a couple of times can make your cravings diminish. Get out for a walk or run, you could get a smartwatch that helps you calculate your heart rate and calorie burn and enjoy the process while you are at it. In case you're stuck at home or workplace, attempt squats, profound knee twists, pushups, running set up, or strolling all over a bunch of steps. If actual work doesn't intrigue you, attempt petition, embroidery, woodwork or journaling. Energy burn has a way to stimulate your brain to enjoy a healthy ride.

CHAPTER FOUR
Think Positive

Thinking is the first thing we do when we wake up, simply owning to the fact that we must make decisions once we wake up every morning or day for those who have a different sleeping cycle. Do you know it is very possible to be the most positive thinker on earth, yet come up with the worst decisions or act badly? This happens because of our limited nature as humans, we are not perfect, but through consistency and truthfulness, we could work harder to achieve our goals in life and mend our broken paths. In this chapter let us x-ray the pattern of thoughts that creates the good, bad, and favourable habits.

Smoking addiction is not safe, as a lot of things could go wrong, I once watched a movie whereby a cigarette caused a high impact explosion. I know what it looks like to be with a cycle of bad habits, it looks like it just would not stop, what you need to do henceforth is try these positive thinking methods below.

Mind-body sync: It is helpful to know that the first step to getting what you want is knowing that there are possibilities in limited moments. Our body and mind are in sync with our thoughts, for instance, you want to change the interior design of your house you don't just think about it, see it and leave it, you have to bring financial and human resources to accomplish the set goal. The same way having control over an addiction begins, it has to be in sync with your mind, body and soul to completely break out from that control. Yes, you can quit smoking when your mind and body are in control. You could start with things that are easier for you to control then you advance to the harder parts. Let me say the little things to quit smoking could be knowing the triggers while the harder parts could be having control and avoiding the triggers. Create a mental guide that helps you control your mind and body to accept your decision to quit smoking.

Self-Decision: In quitting smoking, you have to first make a self-decision to break the habit. The 'self' in the decision means that you have realized that smoking as a habit is what you want to get rid of. This means that the decision is not forced but self-motivated. The self-motivation in this propels positive thinking which is what you need in starting out to break that smoking habit. Think of the good old days without smoking, the days of good accomplishment and things that brought joy to you. As you're starting out on stopping smoking, you focus on the decision to quit smoking; think of moments that give you reliefs apart from smoking time; make notes of your daily changes on the decision; play or watch fun movies/audios; join a group of friends who make you happy; talk positively to yourself on the decision and identify your weaknesses. Thinking positive has been proven to reduce stress which is a leading factor for complicity in morbidity resulting from smoking. Remember you have to think positively about yourself, and your decision as a sustenance to yielding results from your efforts on breaking the smoking habit.

CHAPTER FIVE
Get Moving

It's not just about deciding to quit, it's about remaining committed to your work-out personal plans to quit. You need to remember that you made a self-decision to stop smoking; it's neither forced nor compelled on you. The self-decision should be a drive that keeps you going on the journey to renege smoking. When you decide to quit smoking, you have set in actions certain feelings in you will struggle with the existing feelings of pleasure that comes from smoking. This positions you in a tight corner where you might have to pick between staying healthy without smoking or satisfying your hormone-pushed desires to get pleasure by lighting the next cigarette. Just like Nelson Mandela said, "It always seems impossible until it's done." This explains that it may appear impossible at first until you stay off smoking the first day, then the second, third week, months and years. To keep moving on your decision to quit smoking:

Make the decision to quit a goal: The contrast between a goal and an objective is action or reality. Defining feasible objectives for yourself is a basic and dreary course toward bigger or more yearning objectives. Goal setting requires both accomplishment and disappointment, so it's critical to value both while developing your quit smoking plan. A New Year's goal is just one little advance over a wish; it's an aim with an obscure or non-existent arrangement, and without documentation could result in a mere wish. To quit smoking within the time frame of 30 days is a more realistic plan that needs to be documented every single day.

Short-term goal to long-term goal: Goal setting requires an ideal outcome and could be basically characterized as the way toward choosing what to achieve, defining an objective is that we want some specific things to happen, thereby the need for change in our daily routine is paramount. Goal setting from short term to long term is the best quit smoking plan needed to get ready for the future and accomplish some similarity to our current dreams. Let this be your mantra: Time to move on to better things. Eliminate all that has to do with smoking; lighters, ashtrays, even the dashboard lighter in your vehicle. Smell new rather than smoky.

Organize your routines: Knowing why you need to stop can help you stay inspired. Do you desire to be more dynamic, to look and feel good, or to bring down your odds of a drawn-out sickness? Whatever the explanation may be, it's your explanation, as it's the most significant. Prepare a follow-up routine that interests you, ensure to put your smoking mantra or logo that would help you get moving on your quit smoking plan.

Motivate yourself to stay committed: Have faith in yourself – This is basic! Stay positive and put hope in yourself and what you are achieving. Create a timetable with steps on how you will arrive at your objective. Set cut-off times for each progression and cross them off as you achieve every one of them on your list. Be adaptable – Remember that difficulties can occur. Try not to get frustrated and surrender. Continue trying constantly!

Consider the long term effect of staying off smoking: The most important thing you need to think of is your health. The goal should be creating and maintaining a healthy lifestyle that is sustainable and enjoyable. Smoking changes the internal structure of the heart and lungs due to the release of chemicals ingested into the body through smoking. Staying off smoking reduces the risk of heart attack, dull memory, breathing problems, mouth odour and several other health-related problems.

Be truthful to yourself: The word truth can be termed a good virtue. When it comes to creating good habits you have to own your truth. There is a difference between a deliberate act to change a bad habit and leaving in self-denial of a bad habit, the process of change and self-denial could be the reason why a quit smoking plan might be easier to achieve or difficult to actualize. You need to be truthful to yourself on the reasons why you started smoking and create the best escape route. Only you can help yourself completely quit smoking.

Make the quit process gradual: The best strategy to adopt is withdrawal symptoms. A day is enough to resist the urge to smoking, gradually reduce the quantity then let the feeling fade till you perfect your quit smoking plan. The best way to introduce addiction changes is by practising gradual reduction, this would help your mind and body prepare for the bigger goal.

Timely evaluate your commitment to stop smoking: Personal assessment is vital for your quit smoking plan, this would set the ball rolling from desired to expected results. Some metrics you can use to evaluate your plans are; focus, cravings, smoking reduction, anxiety, irritability, appetite and weight gain. I went for a seminar some years back and I was opportune to hear from people who were having a hard time quitting smoking, A man told us he used to smoke 40 cigarettes in a day and today he is a zero free smoker, he was able to achieve it through a timer he had on his phone that helped him monitor his daily activities. I strongly believe that there is a strategy that works for everyone no matter how deep or bad a smoking addiction could be, evaluate your progress and keep up being positive about your situation, you would eventually reach your set goals.

CHAPTER SIX
Your Personal Quit Smoking Plan

Just as we create our daily routine for meals, career, work, business, family or relationships we could also create a mental and physical guide to help us cope with addictions. The fact that smoking is hard to quit should compel us to consider the deadly resultants such as: high blood pressure, cancer, respiratory disorders, chronic heart diseases, diabetes and other deadly infections. Quitting is the antidote to the deadliness of smoking. This is why you need a personal plan on how to quit smoking that can always be with you all the time. You need to know that within the first 10 seconds of a puff, harmful chemicals are released into you and they penetrate your lungs, brain, heart and flow through your blood wreaking havoc on your body system. This identifies how fast the harm can be and why you need a personalized plan to quit smoking. Follow as we roll out the plans together.

The goal of this book is to help people, the best way to help others is by sharing true-life experiences of people who have gone through similar experiences so that through their paths we could see possibilities why copying with our own situations. Why undergoing research for this book, I came across the success story of Eugennie Mercredi shared on her quit smoking story, she emphasized how she strengthened her willpower to make the quit smoking plan possible. Eugennie had high blood pressure but decided to go on a journey of quitting smoking. Although she worked as a health promoter in Canada, smoking had become a part of her but she later decided to be a figure to model in preaching healthy living. This impulsed her decision to quit smoking. Her personal plans for quitting included: eating healthy, going for a walk with hubby instead of smoking, and daily monitoring the progress on staying off cigarette.

As a personal plan to quit smoking, you should:

Go on a date: Just like you set a date for an important program, you should select a date to quit smoking. Selecting a date makes you see the decision to quit as significant. Make this quit smoking date fun, enjoyable and memorable, yes you need to enjoy the process, it is about time. You must decide to gradually stop smoking or effect the quit on the selected date. Please note that there could likely be an immersion into the habit, it is better to gradually stop smoking – a continuous drop can make a waterway. On the chosen day, medical experts have advised that it is functional to have informed a friend or colleague about the decision, put away cigarettes and ashtrays, develop a support system or evaluate your previous quit trial to inform the latter decision. Then, you should do this: Delay your craving to smoke to have it go down; take a deep breath to have a rush in of fresh air into your lungs; drink water to calm yourself; get a task done to keep yourself busy. It is important to ensure that you start on the set date. Procrastination can only make matters worse- don't indulge.

Go the NRT way: This formula NRT is widely known as Nicotine replacement therapy it's possible to quit smoking but difficult to sustain and be without nicotine.

This difficulty is high especially if one has become addicted to smoking. To have nicotine released into the body in a harmless way, NRT can be used. The cravings for cigarette and tobacco becomes reduced when an alternative source of nicotine is introduced to the body. Research on smoking shows that using nicotine replacement therapy (NRT) can in about 15-36% increase the high chances of quitting smoking, especially when combined with gum or lozenge.

Adopt non-nicotine medications: If you don't want to get nicotine involved at all, you can talk to your doctor about your decision to use non-nicotine medications to help in quitting smoking. There are two main medications approved by the FDA for non-nicotine use to include Bupropion; which works in the brain to lessen the desire for nicotine and Varenicline; which works in reducing the level of pleasure you derive from nicotine and its withdrawal symptoms.

Engage in behavioural support: This proves functional when you combine behavioural support with NRT or even the non-nicotine medications. What you get is the right support that helps you be more in control of your responses to stimuli. By behavioural support, you can have your counsellor offer you materials, explanations and approaches to make your decision to quit smoking successful.

CHAPTER SEVEN
Foods to Help Quit Smoking

A healthy eating routine is very important for any individual that is keen on their quit smoking plan. Fruits and vegetables are a good alternative to munch on to help you control the craving of always wanting to put something in your mouth. Grains, lean protein sources, dairy or other calcium sources, nuts, seeds, and olive oil are a good option for you to consider. Smoking dulls the ability to taste and smell. Stay away from Alcohol, high fat, sugar, sodium, and calories when you're attempting to stop smoking. Healthy food or drink can fill the very same need smoking does.

A few food sources can build your odds of remaining smoke-free for great. Smoking influences your feeling of taste, you may find that food begins to taste in an unexpected way. This might be an extraordinary chance to attempt healthy nourishments to discover a few things you like.

The right combination of food can help stimulate your decision to stay off smoking. American Heart Association through research recommends that foods in the following combination help when quitting smoking:

Healthy Snacks: This could come in form of ready to eat snacks, some good options to consider are the following: whole-wheat or bagel, whole-grain muffin, fruits (apple, banana, peach), low-fat yoghurt, whole-grain cereal, unsalted nuts.

DIY healthy eats: Just go into your kitchen and try out some easy recipe with few ingredients, you could try out these easy to make eats: Sandwich, vegetables (carrots, celery, cucumbers, and green peppers), fruits (watermelon, pineapple), popcorn, and smoothie.

Emergency foods: Food is essential, it is good to eat healthy. Take time in your meal prep to create an emergency food plan. Here are some options to consider: vegetables (carrots, celery, cucumbers, and green peppers), no sugar gum, no sugar candy or mints.

Frozen treats: Sometimes your mouth needs something that's unique, I would recommend frozen treats some great options could be: frozen banana, juice bars, sugarless sherbet, less calorie ice cream, low-fat yoghurt.

Having these foods close to you helps you have alternatives ready. Instead of smoking, you can help yourself with fruits, vegetables and frozen treats that also give you pleasure while keeping you healthy always.

CHAPTER EIGHT
Preventing Weight Gain after You Stop Smoking

The common assumption people with smoking addiction have is the fear of 'weight gain.' that could come when they eventually quit smoking. This is why people ask mostly when they are on the verge of deciding to quit or not to quit; will I gain weight? Experts affirm that although people who quit smoking may nurture the fear of weight gain when they quit, studies have shown that rather than gain weight, people shed calories when they embark on smoking cessation. Instead of relying on nicotine to boost your metabolism and maintain your weight, you can naturally keep fit by engaging in physical exercises which make you maintain not only your body but also a healthy lifestyle. After deciding to quit smoking, you should remember to revive your sporting life and stay active naturally all the time without lifting a cigarette or releasing a puff.

Appetite Control: Mindful eating is key to quitting smoking. Keep your weight in check by first doing a belly check, then plan towards reducing your calorie intake, consider being aware of the foods you eat daily, after which you reduce your portion intake. Start gradually then improve on your appetite control. When you quit smoking, you may feel hungrier and eat more than you used to, ensure you stay hydrated. It will hold you back from eating when you really desire to. Adding more protein to your eating regimen can build sensations of completion, cause you want to eat less at your next supper, this can assist you with losing fat. You could consider animal or plant-based protein sources to satisfy your cravings. Animal protein gives all fundamental amino acids in the right proportion, you could get them from meat, fish, eggs, or dairy consistently, you would probably get sufficient protein from these options. For plant-based protein Lentils are good supplements. Seitan is also another good source of plant-based protein, it is produced using wheat gluten. Soybean can be used to make the following plant-based protein sources: Tofu, tempeh, and edamame. Beans are well-being advancing, protein-pressed vegetables that contain an assortment of nutrients, minerals, and advantageous plant compounds. Also, take more normal grains.

Exercise Regularly: Smoking in a way might help you burn some calories but in the long run, the health effects are very dangerous. What you need is a healthy plan to help you increase your metabolism and control the weight gain that might come after you quit smoking. It could be difficult to stick to an exercise routine, especially for those who desire to quit smoking completely. First, you struggle then you commit and it eventually gets better. Making exercise a pleasant piece of your regular daily existence might be simpler than you might suspect. You don't need to go through repetitive or difficult exercises adding active work to your weekly schedule can profoundly affect your wellbeing. Self-empathy improves the probability that you'll succeed. Try not to complain about your body, your present wellness level, or your alleged absence of self-control. Daily workout could help you keep fit when trying to quit smoking. Get into any event that consists of 150 minutes of moderate oxygen-consuming action or 75 minutes of incredible high-impact movement seven days, or a mix of moderate and lively action. Try some aerobic activities or strength training such as: walking, skipping, running, jogging, swimming, cardio kickboxing, Zumba fitness, cycling, squats, push-ups, plank, yoga poses and several others that you might find interesting.

Avoid Distractions: A lot of things are happening in our daily lives, most times it's difficult to escape from distractions that could come from our phone, television, computer, environment, work, family, friends and other areas of our existence. When you want to completely quit smoking it is crucial to understand that distractions needs to be under check as some of them could be a link to smoking triggers. For a complete quit smoking plan to work effectively please stay away from every form of smoking cravings or tempting situations, rather than smoking, pick up a good habit of saving the money you would normally use to buy cigarettes invest in a good cause; try investing that money in stocks or cryptocurrency. Make a list of 10 things that could distract you and 10 things that could inspire you to keep up with your quit smoking plan. After you might have made your 10 lists of distractions and inspirations, do a cross match and figure out how you could replace distractions with inspirations and at the end of the week do an audit to see how your journey went? Always remember you are in control of your life. There is something we always forget to do when trying to come out of a bad habit, this could be tricky but isolation is one of the reasons why quitting bad habits is unattainable. Isolation could make us unaccountable, therefore seeing or hearing from someone who shares the same goal to quit smoking could help you become more accountable. There was a time when I had a serious craving and I immediately ran outside to where people were discussing, I only stayed there for 5 minutes and the trigger disappeared. Distractions may not just come from external forms, sometimes distractions could come from loneliness and a lot of thoughts begins to fly in and out of our mind.

CHAPTER NINE
What to Do if You Slip or Relapse

As humans, it is possible to desire an end to a habit, try out methods to break the habit and still have the habit bouncing back all time like a rolling ball. It's easy to decide, set a date to quit smoking but it's more demanding to effect the actual stoppage of smoking. It takes well-defined intention and readiness to stay devoted to your resolve to quit smoking. When you feel like returning to smoking, longing for the sensation of pleasure in nicotine, it's that time you have to remind yourself of your decision to quit. Tell yourself, "I don't do this anymore. I have stopped this." Self-talking in this context reminds you of the efforts that you have put in making sure you successfully stop smoking. You have to revisit your plans and note the dark areas in working on your decision. When you identify the weakness, then you can build on it when making the next resolve to quit smoking.

Some life coach or therapists preach this encouraging message "don't start smoking." Meaning never start what is hard to finish or live by, this is an expression propelled by the arduousness people face before they finally quit smoking. Your personal quit smoking plan could be to stop when married or when you get a better paying job or in the near future, whichever plan you decide on remember today could mark the beginning of your quit smoking plan. Yes, your decision to quit smoking could work. This is a short story of Alfred; while outside one day for a video relaxation, he was on the wait, while there, he received a cigarette from the person sitting next to him. That solo smoking experience reactivated all his cravings for smoking. He went on a non-stop smoking for five months before evaluating his decisions and finally making a resolve to cede from smoking. The story of Alfred affirms that it is possible to relapse after deciding to break the smoking habit but picking up yourself to try again, this time gradually and strategically will eventually create a win situation.

What could go wrong? Relapse is not the worst decision, the very worst is when you give up on yourself. Never give up on your quit smoking plan, with dedication, self-love, active and conscious efforts everything would come into a perfect plan and triggers and relapse would become a thing of the past. Recognize when your mind is drifting. Before a smoking relapse would occur the triggers comes before the actual event takes place. Before we take any actions our mind must have played or relayed the message to our brain before we partake in the activity. It is worthy of note to understand that smoking relapse could occur with a shift in thinking, this might start with something as simple as seeing someone smoking a cigarette during your leisure time. You could think you have quit smoking so the action of the stranger smoking should not bother you, this is when you need to remember that anything could go wrong and a relapse could occur. Two things could lead to a relapse, the first being an unconscious mind in a triggered environment while the other could be forgetting to unclutter your mind from passive triggers. A self-aware individual is always conscious of events happening around their environment, but an unconscious mind tends to blend into whatever is happening within the environment, which in the long run could exhibit some unconscious habits or traits. Have you ever wondered why you hear some parents say to their children? I wonder where you picked this habit from? The truth is that we have things going on in our environment that could form habits or traits associated with us. A lot of things could go wrong when we are not paying close attention, or let things slide. At this point, you might have quit smoking but never forget a relapse could go wrong, keep your zero smoking plan and activities alive and accountable.

Stay Strong: There are days when it seems very difficult to overlook smoking triggers and anxiety or restlessness sets in, this is what you must remember, stay strong to overcome all obstacles and take full control of your mind and body. You can in any case avoid smoking relapse remind yourself why you need to stop. At that point take control once more. Try not to get sad about the relapse, set another quit date, possibly in a week or somewhere within a short time frame. Learn from what made you go into a relapse and find better ways that would help you abstain from smoking in the coming days. Work on your adapting abilities so you're set up whenever you're in a similar circumstance. Stay positive, Keep in mind you would be more grounded in the future since you have realized what to pay special attention to. Nobody is above mistakes, stay strong and overcome your fear of smoking relapse. Never underestimate the need to seek professional help from trained professionals at (social care and support) NHS Smokefree helpline. Kindly visit their website or call for further help as they could also help you overcome your fear of relapse or quit smoking completely. There are many possibilities for you to quit smoking completely it could happen faster than you know it, even when it takes time never give up keep working towards a smoke-free life.

CHAPTER TEN
Helping a Loved One to Stop Smoking

One of the ways to exude true friendship or display love is to help a loved one quit smoking. You know it's not enough to capitalize on "smokers are liable to die young". What matters is how you assist the smoker who is in need of help to break that habit. It's easier said than done to stop a habit. However, by following the how-to provided in this book, you can conquer without a surge to return to the old habit of smoking.

You might not understand what it means to struggle with smoking addiction, but you can encourage or create a working list of how you can help a loved one quit smoking. The following guide below should help you teach or help someone close to you find an escape route from smoking.

Identify with them: You could help them by sharing true stories of how you were able to overcome a bad habit, by this, you show that you understand what they are experiencing and their trials to break the habit. Talk to them about how much could have been saved if smoking isn't involved, and remind them of the fact that you want to always see them with you. Soothing words resonate in breaking bad habits. There is something I tell people who are struggling with a habit they desire to quit, never give up on yourself the bad would become good it only takes patience. Never judge people fighting their battle with smoking addiction, tell them that they are on their way to self-recovery and you wish them the best on their journey to a smoke-free life.

Assist them: There are several things you could do to help others find the needed help they have been thinking of. Some kind acts could be helping with some smoke-free activities, you could also help them get the prescribed drugs as recommended by their doctors after deciding to quit. You can get rid of packs of cigarette and ashtrays within the house and help them avoid places where smoking spree is, to prevent them from being triggered again. Just show a little help to your loved one that is trying to quit smoking, you never know you could feature in their biography someday when they look back at their struggles and consider how far they have come.

Exercise patience in helping them: Some reactions follow the cessation of smoking. It's not easy to reject a pleasure-inducing habit. This is why restlessness, sleeping difficulties, irritations, anger and anxiety can become attached when they withdraw from smoking, try to understand their plight and don't do anything to make them feel unworthy of love or kindness. Be patient with your loved ones trying to quit smoking because they are in a phase that determines if they would fully recover and stay green or they would relapse and get worse, a lot of things could happen, so please mind your words and actions around them.

Engage them: Do you know some people's love language is quality time? Yes sometimes love has a way of helping people recover very quickly. You can help your loved ones trying to quit smoking get busy to take their mind away from their smoking addiction. When you notice they're becoming fixed on issues around tobacco or cigarette, remind them of an assignment and why they need to meet the schedule. Engage them in activities that would help them get rewarded in their career, finance, academics, health, relationship or other areas of their life.

Remember to do it in love: There is a universal language that unites or binds hearts across the world, it is called love. A lot of problems in the world would cease if we truly love, respect and tolerate each other. Helping a loved one quit smoking has to be done in love, of cause we know some virtues of love should exhibit the following: patience, kindness, gentleness, commitment, friendship, quality time and several others. Love conquers all things, do good to people and they would become better. Live, love, learn and forgive. Never run out of love, one good turn can change someone's life around.

CONCLUSION

Because pleasure comes from smoking, the brain becomes conditioned to wanting it all the time. A smoker can go from a single cigarette in a day to smoking packs in hours. In the economics of smoking, the longer the habit becomes, the higher the number of smoked substances becomes. It's important to note that it is easy to express the willingness to quit smoking, but having a personal guide on how-to, as in this book makes it all possible to stop smoking.

One step at a time: At first it might seem very difficult to let go of smoking addiction but with consistency and self-love you can overcome every hurdle you think is impossible, get started and live a clean and healthier life.

Believe in you: When it comes to the will to quit smoking addictions it is in your control to determine what goes on in your life, you have the power to say no to a pattern you do not wish to continue.

Know your triggers: Never ignore the signs it comes way before the smoking activity happens. Be conscious of your mind, environment, what you hear and see. Never be caught unaware by smoking addiction know when to put things in control.

References

[1] Santos-Longhurst, A. (2019). Benefits of thinking positively, and how to do it https://www.heaalthline.com/health/how-to-think-positive

[2] American Heart Association (2018). Why is it so hard to quit smoking https://www.heart.org/en/news/2018/10/17/why-its-so-hard-to-quit-smoking

[3] Jaffe, A. (2019). Why is it so hard to change bad https://www.google.com/amp/s/www.psychologytoday.com/us/blog/all-about-addiction/201903/why-is-it-so-hard-change-bad-habits%3famp

[4] Australian Government Department of Health. What are the effects of smoking and tobacco https://www.health.gov.au/health-topics/smoking-and-tobacco/about-smoking-and-tobcco/what-are-the-effects-of-smoking-and-tobacco

[5] Eugennie, M. –Breathe the Lung Association https://www.lung.ca/ling-health/smoking-and-tobacco/quitting-success/eugennie-mercredi

[6] Nichols, H. (2017). Five ways to quit smoking https://www.google.com/amp/s/www.medicalnewstoday.com/amp/articles/319460

[7] Robinson, J. (2019). Combination NRT linked to higher smoking quit rate than single forms https://pharmaceuticals-journal.com/article/news/combination-nrt-linked-to-higher-smoking-quit-rate-than-single-forms

[8] Smoking triggers https://www.healthlinkbc.ca/health-topics/99152863

[9] Weatherspoon, D. (2018). Everything you need to know about nicotine https://www.medicalnewstoday.com/articles/240820

[10] Ken, W. – Breathe the Lung Association https://www.lung.ca/lung-health/smoking-and-tobacco/quitting-success/ken-wareham-st-johns-nfld

[11] American Heart Association/Nicotinell. What to eat when quitting smoking https://www.nicotinell.co.uk/how-to-quit-smoking/starting-your-quit-smoking/what-to-eat.html

[12] Matthews Internal Medicine. The connection between smoking cessation and weight loss https:/matthewsmd.com/news/connection-smoking-cessation-weight-loss/#:-:text=For%20many%20people%2C%20quitting%20smoking,according%20to20a%20recent%20study

[13] Reginald M. – Breath the Lung Association https://www.lung.ca/lung-health/smoking-and-tobacco/quitting-success/reginald-mercredi

[14] Goodwin, M. (2021). Help your partner quit smoking https://www.healthline.com/health/quit-smoking-spouse

www.ingramcontent.com/pod-product-compliance
Lightning Source LLC
Chambersburg PA
CBHW070310220526
45465CB00004B/1831